LEAKY GUT COOKBOOK

DR. KIMBERLY CARLOS

TABLE OF CONTENT

INTRODUCTION

Once upon a time, in a quiet suburban neighborhood, lived a woman named Sarah. She had always been full of life and energy until a mysterious ailment took its toll on her. Sarah was diagnosed with a condition known as "leaky gut," a disorder that left her feeling constantly fatigued, bloated, and in discomfort. She visited doctors, tried various medications, and underwent numerous tests, but nothing seemed to provide lasting relief.

One day, frustrated with her condition and determined to take control of her health, Sarah embarked on a journey of self-discovery. She delved deep into research about leaky gut and how dietary changes could potentially help. She spent countless hours reading books, articles, and consulting with holistic health practitioners.

Armed with knowledge, Sarah transformed her kitchen into a haven of wholesome ingredients. She embraced a diet rich in whole foods, focusing on gut-healing options like bone broth, fermented vegetables, and anti-inflammatory herbs and spices. She bid farewell to processed foods, gluten, dairy, and sugar, which she had learned could exacerbate her condition.

As the weeks turned into months, Sarah noticed subtle changes. Her energy levels began to rise, her bloating reduced, and her overall sense of well-being improved. The road to recovery was not without its challenges, as she faced cravings and moments of doubt, but her determination never wavered.

Sarah's friends and family marveled at her transformation. They watched in awe as her radiant health returned, and her laughter echoed once more. She felt like her old self again, thanks to the incredible power of a well-balanced, gut-nourishing diet.

Over time, Sarah's story inspired others facing similar health challenges. She shared her knowledge and experiences, helping them take the first steps towards healing their own leaky guts. Sarah's journey was a testament to the remarkable healing potential of the right diet, illustrating that sometimes, the path to wellness begins with the choices we make in our own kitchens.

CHAPTER ONE

Leaky Gut: Types, Causes and Symptoms

Leaky gut syndrome, also known as increased intestinal permeability, is a condition that has gained attention in recent years for its potential role in various health issues. It involves a compromised intestinal barrier, which can allow undigested food particles, toxins, and bacteria to leak from the gut into the bloodstream, triggering immune responses and inflammation.

While the medical community is still exploring the full scope of leaky gut, there are several types, causes, and symptoms associated with this condition.

Types of Leaky Gut

1. Primary Leaky Gut: This is the most common type, characterized by an impaired intestinal barrier due to factors such as diet, stress, and medication use.

2. Secondary Leaky Gut: Often caused by underlying conditions like celiac disease, Crohn's disease, or irritable bowel syndrome (IBS), secondary leaky gut results from the inflammation and damage associated with these diseases.

Causes of Leaky Gut

1. Dietary Factors: A diet high in processed foods, refined sugars, gluten, and dairy can contribute to intestinal inflammation and permeability.

2. Chronic Stress: Prolonged stress can weaken the gut lining, making it more susceptible to damage.

3. Medications: Certain medications, such as nonsteroidal anti-inflammatory drugs (NSAIDs) and antibiotics, can disrupt the gut microbiota and contribute to leaky gut.

4. Infections: Bacterial, viral, or parasitic infections can damage the intestinal lining, leading to increased permeability.

5. Environmental Toxins: Exposure to pollutants and environmental toxins can have a detrimental effect on the gut **barrier.**

6. Genetic Predisposition: Some individuals may be genetically more susceptible to developing leaky gut.

Symptoms of Leaky Gut

1. Digestive Issues: This includes chronic diarrhea, constipation, bloating, and gas.

2. Food Sensitivities: Individuals with leaky gut may become sensitive to certain foods, experiencing adverse reactions upon consumption.

3. Nutritional Deficiencies: Malabsorption due to a compromised gut can lead to deficiencies in vitamins and minerals.

4. Autoimmune Conditions: There is a link between leaky gut and autoimmune diseases, as the immune system may react to substances that leak into the bloodstream.

5. Fatigue: Chronic fatigue is a common symptom, as the body expends extra energy combating inflammation.

6. Skin Problems: Conditions like acne, eczema, and psoriasis may worsen or be triggered by leaky gut.

7. Mood Disorders: Some individuals may experience anxiety, depression, or mood swings, as the gut-brain connection is disrupted.

8. Joint Pain: Joint inflammation and pain can be associated with leaky gut.

Following a Leaky Gut Diet with Benefits

Following a leaky gut diet can potentially help improve gut health and alleviate symptoms associated with increased intestinal permeability.

While there is no one-size-fits-all approach, as individual reactions to foods vary, here are some general guidelines for adopting a leaky gut diet along with its benefits:

1. Remove Inflammatory Foods:

- Gluten:Eliminate or significantly reduce gluten-containing grains like wheat, barley, and rye. Gluten can contribute to inflammation in the gut.
- Dairy:Avoid or limit dairy products, as lactose and casein can be problematic for some individuals.
- Processed Foods:Minimize consumption of processed and packaged foods, which often contain additives, preservatives, and unhealthy fats that may worsen gut inflammation.

2. Emphasize Gut-Healing Foods:

-   Bone Broth:Rich in collagen and amino acids, bone broth can support gut lining repair.
-   Fermented Foods:Incorporate probiotic-rich foods like sauerkraut, kimchi, yogurt (if tolerated), and kefir to promote a healthy gut microbiome.
-   Omega-3 Fatty Acids:Consume foods high in omega-3s, such as fatty fish (salmon, mackerel), flaxseeds, and walnuts, to reduce inflammation.

3. Eat Fiber-Rich Foods: Incorporate plenty of fiber from fruits, vegetables, and whole grains (if tolerated). Fiber supports beneficial gut bacteria and helps maintain regular bowel movements.

4. Anti-Inflammatory Spices and Herbs: Use turmeric, ginger, garlic, and other herbs and spices with anti-inflammatory properties to season your meals.

5. Consider Supplements: Consult with a healthcare provider or registered dietitian about supplements like L-glutamine, quercetin, and digestive enzymes, which may support gut healing.

6. Hydration: Drink plenty of water to keep the mucosal lining of the intestines hydrated and functioning optimally.

7. Manage Stress: Practice stress management techniques like meditation, yoga, or deep breathing exercises, as chronic stress can contribute to gut issues.

8. Gradual Introduction of Foods: If you suspect specific foods trigger symptoms, try reintroducing them one at a time in small quantities to identify and avoid problematic items.

Benefits of Following a Leaky Gut Diet

1. Reduced Inflammation: A well-balanced leaky gut diet can help reduce gut inflammation, which is often at the root of many health issues.

2. Improved Digestion: Avoiding problematic foods and including gut-friendly choices can lead to better digestion and fewer digestive symptoms.

3. Enhanced Nutrient Absorption: A healthier gut lining allows for improved absorption of essential nutrients, reducing the risk of nutritional deficiencies.

4. Balanced Gut Microbiome: Consuming probiotic-rich foods can support a diverse and balanced gut microbiome, which is crucial for overall health.

5. Symptom Relief: Many individuals experience relief from symptoms like bloating, gas, diarrhea, and fatigue when following a leaky gut diet tailored to their needs.

6. Support for Autoimmune Conditions: Some people with autoimmune conditions report improvements in symptoms by adopting a gut-friendly diet.

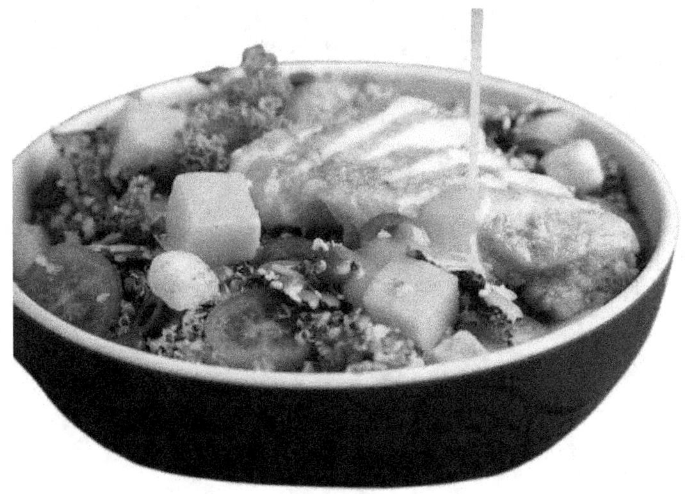

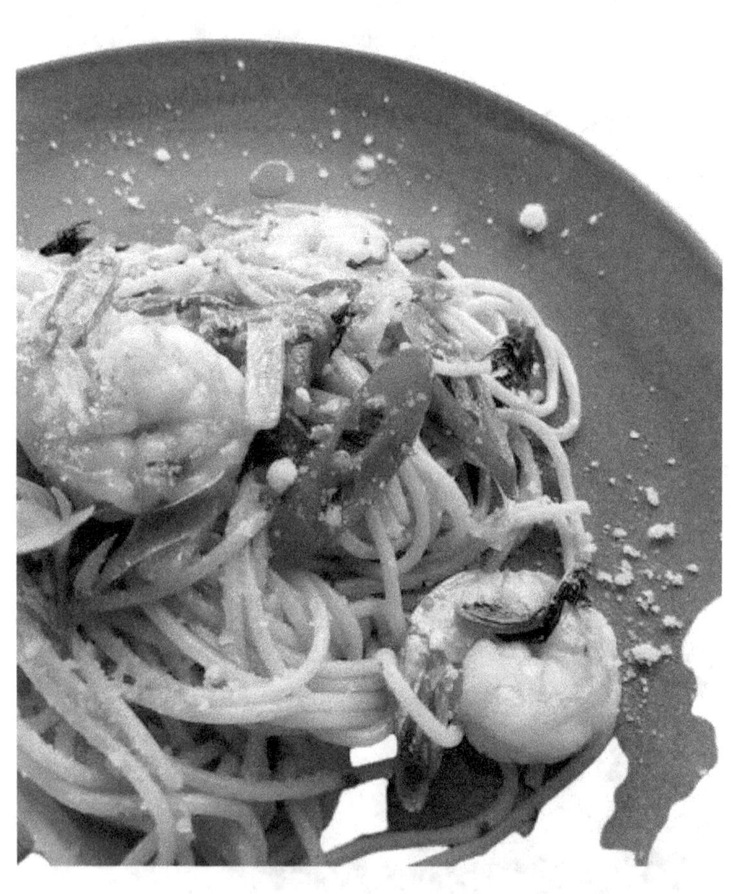

CHAPTER TWO

14-Day Meal Plan For Leaky Gut

Day 1

Breakfast:

- Scrambled eggs with spinach and avocado.
- A cup of ginger tea.

Lunch:

- Grilled chicken breast with a side of steamed broccoli.
- Quinoa salad with cucumber, cherry tomatoes, and lemon-tahini dressing.

Snack:

- Carrot sticks with hummus.

Dinner:

- Baked salmon with asparagus and a side of mashed sweet potatoes.

Day 2

Breakfast:

- Greek yogurt (if tolerated) with honey and blueberries.
- A small serving of mixed nuts.

Lunch:

- Mixed greens salad with grilled shrimp, cherry tomatoes, and avocado. Dress with olive oil and lemon.

Snack:

- Sliced cucumber and radish with guacamole.

Dinner:

- Turkey and vegetable stir-fry with cauliflower rice.

Day 3

Breakfast:

- Smoothie with spinach, banana, almond milk, and a scoop of collagen powder.

Lunch:

- Lentil and vegetable soup.

- A small side salad with olive oil and vinegar.

Snack:

- Sliced apple with almond butter.

Dinner:

- Baked cod with roasted Brussels sprouts and quinoa.

Day 4

Breakfast:

- Oatmeal (gluten-free if necessary) topped with sliced strawberries and a drizzle of honey.

Lunch:

- Grilled chicken and vegetable kebabs with a side of brown rice.

Snack:

- Celery sticks with almond cream cheese.

Dinner:

- Beef and vegetable stew with a side of steamed green beans.

Day 5

Breakfast:

- Scrambled eggs with sautéed spinach, mushrooms, and a sprinkle of nutritional yeast.

Lunch:

- Tuna salad with mixed greens, cherry tomatoes, and a lemon-tahini dressing.

Snack:

- Mixed berries (blueberries, raspberries, strawberries).

Dinner:

- Baked chicken thighs with roasted carrots and

quinoa.

Day 6

Breakfast:

- Smoothie with kale, banana, almond milk, and a
  spoonful of chia seeds.

Lunch:

- Grilled salmon with a side of steamed asparagus and
  mashed cauliflower.

Snack:

- Sliced bell peppers with guacamole.

Dinner:

- Pork tenderloin with sautéed zucchini and a side of
  brown rice.

Day 7

Breakfast:

- Overnight chia pudding made with almond milk,
  topped with sliced peaches and a sprinkle of

cinnamon.

Lunch:

- Quinoa and black bean salad with diced avocado, red onion, and cilantro.

Snack:

- A handful of mixed nuts.

Dinner:

- Turkey and vegetable meatballs served with spaghetti squash and marinara sauce (check for added sugar).

Day 8

Breakfast:

- Scrambled eggs with sautéed spinach and a side of sliced avocado.

Lunch:

- Grilled chicken breast with roasted sweet potatoes and a side of mixed greens.

Snack:

- Sliced cucumber and carrot sticks with hummus.

Dinner:

- Baked cod with a side of steamed broccoli and quinoa.

Day 9

Breakfast:

- Greek yogurt (if tolerated) with honey, raspberries, and a sprinkle of ground flaxseeds.

Lunch:

- Spinach and roasted beet salad with grilled shrimp and a balsamic vinaigrette.

Snack:

- Sliced pear with almond butter.

Dinner:

- Turkey and vegetable stir-fry with cauliflower rice.

Day 10

Breakfast:

- Smoothie with spinach, banana, almond milk, and a
  scoop of collagen powder.

Lunch:

- Lentil and vegetable soup with a side of mixed
  greens.

Snack:

- Sliced bell peppers with guacamole.

Dinner:

- Baked chicken thighs with roasted Brussels sprouts
  and quinoa.

Day 11

Breakfast:

- Oatmeal (gluten-free if necessary) with sliced
  strawberries and a drizzle of honey.

Lunch:

- Grilled chicken and vegetable kebabs with a side of brown rice.

Snack:

- Celery sticks with almond cream cheese.

Dinner:

- Beef and vegetable stew with a side of steamed green beans.

Day 12

Breakfast:

- Scrambled eggs with sautéed spinach, mushrooms, and a sprinkle of nutritional yeast.

Lunch:

- Tuna salad with mixed greens, cherry tomatoes, and a lemon-tahini dressing.

Snack:

- Mixed berries (blueberries, raspberries,

strawberries).

Dinner:

- Baked salmon with roasted carrots and quinoa.

Day 13

Breakfast:

- Smoothie with kale, banana, almond milk, and a spoonful of chia seeds.

Lunch:

- Grilled pork tenderloin with a side of sautéed zucchini and brown rice.

Snack:

- A handful of mixed nuts.

Dinner:

- Chicken and vegetable stir-fry with broccoli and cauliflower rice.

Day 14

Breakfast:

- Overnight chia pudding made with almond milk, topped with sliced peaches and a sprinkle of cinnamon.

Lunch:

- Quinoa and black bean salad with diced avocado, red onion, and cilantro.

Snack:

- Sliced apple with almond butter.

Dinner:

- Baked tilapia with a side of steamed asparagus and mashed cauliflower.

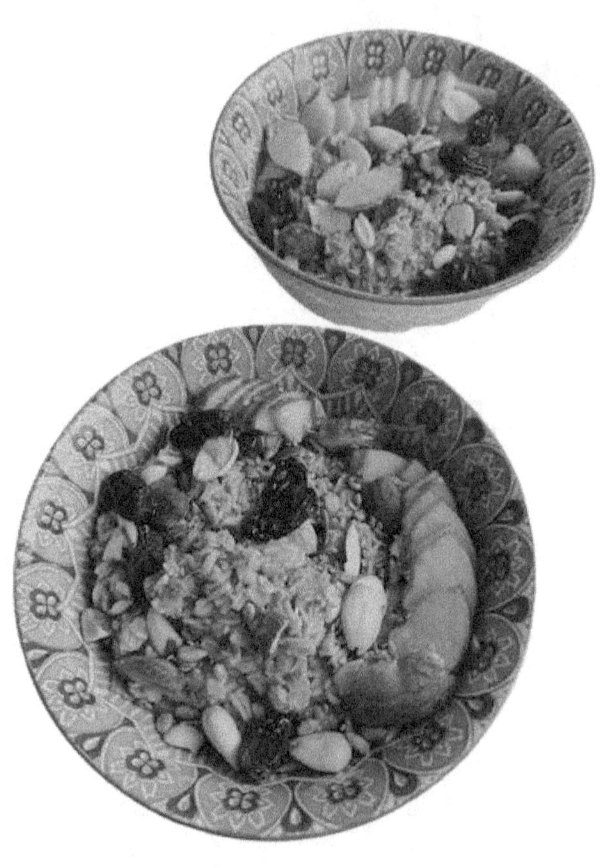

CHAPTER THREE

Leaky Gut Breakfast Recipes

1. Scrambled Eggs with Spinach and Avocado

Ingredients:

- 2 large eggs
- 1 cup fresh spinach leaves
- 1/2 ripe avocado, sliced
- Salt and pepper to taste

Instructions:

1. In a non-stick skillet, heat a little olive oil over medium hcat.

2. Whisk the eggs in a bowl and pour them into the skillet.

3. Add the spinach leaves and scramble until the eggs are cooked to your liking.

4. Season with salt and pepper.

5. Serve with sliced avocado on top.

Cooking Time: 10 minutes

2. Greek Yogurt Parfait

Ingredients:

- 1 cup Greek yogurt (if tolerated)
- 1/2 cup fresh berries (e.g., blueberries, strawberries)
- 1 tablespoon honey or maple syrup (optional)
- 2 tablespoons chopped nuts (e.g., almonds, walnuts)

Instructions:

1. In a glass or bowl, layer Greek yogurt, berries, and a drizzle of honey or maple syrup if desired.

2. Sprinkle with chopped nuts on top.

Cooking Time: 5 minutes

3. Chia Seed Pudding

Ingredients:

- 2 tablespoons chia seeds
- 1 cup almond milk (or any preferred milk)
- 1/2 teaspoon vanilla extract
- Fresh fruit (e.g., sliced bananas, berries) for topping

Instructions:

1. In a jar or bowl, mix chia seeds, almond milk, and vanilla extract.

2. Stir well and refrigerate overnight.

3. In the morning, top with fresh fruit before serving.

Cooking Time: 5 minutes (plus overnight soaking)

4. Green Smoothie

Ingredients:

- 1 cup spinach or kale
- 1/2 banana
- 1/2 cup unsweetened almond milk
- 1 tablespoon almond butter
- 1 scoop collagen powder (optional)

Instructions:

1. Blend all the ingredients until smooth.

2. Add ice cubes if desired.

3. Pour into a glass and enjoy.

Cooking Time: 5 minutes

5. Oatmeal with Berries

Ingredients:

- 1/2 cup gluten-free oats
- 1 cup water or almond milk
- 1/2 cup mixed berries
- 1 tablespoon honey or maple syrup (optional)

Instructions:

1. Cook the oats in water or almond milk according to package instructions.

2. Top with mixed berries and a drizzle of honey or maple syrup if desired.

Cooking Time: 10 minutes

6. Avocado and Smoked Salmon Toast

Ingredients:

- 2 slices gluten-free bread
- 1 ripe avocado, mashed
- 2 ounces smoked salmon
- Sliced cucumber and radish for garnish
- Lemon juice, salt, and pepper to taste

Instructions:

1. Toast the gluten-free bread.

2. Spread mashed avocado on the toast.

3. Top with smoked salmon, sliced cucumber, and radish.

4. Season with lemon juice, salt, and pepper.

Cooking Time: 10 minutes

7. Coconut Yogurt Bowl

Ingredients:

- 1 cup coconut yogurt (dairy-free)
- 1/4 cup granola (gluten-free if necessary)
- Sliced kiwi and mango for topping
- Drizzle of honey (optional)

Instructions:

1. In a bowl, layer coconut yogurt and granola.

2. Top with sliced kiwi and mango.

3. Add a drizzle of honey if desired.

Cooking Time: 5 minutes

8. Sweet Potato Hash

Ingredients:

- 1 small sweet potato, diced
- 1/4 red bell pepper, diced
- 1/4 red onion, diced
- 2 tablespoons olive oil
- Salt, pepper, and paprika to taste

Instructions:

1. Heat olive oil in a skillet over medium heat.

2. Add diced sweet potato, red bell pepper, and red onion.

3. Sauté until the sweet potatoes are tender and slightly crispy.

4. Season with salt, pepper, and paprika.

Cooking Time: 15 minutes

9. Almond Butter Banana Pancakes

Ingredients:

- 2 ripe bananas
- 2 large eggs
- 2 tablespoons almond butter
- 1/2 teaspoon vanilla extract
- 1/4 teaspoon baking powder (gluten-free)
- Sliced bananas and a drizzle of honey for topping

Instructions:

1. In a blender, combine ripe bananas, eggs, almond butter, vanilla extract, and baking powder.

2. Blend until smooth.

3. Heat a non-stick skillet over medium heat and pour small pancake-sized portions of the batter.

4. Cook until bubbles form on the surface, then flip and cook the other side.

5. Top with sliced bananas and a drizzle of honey.

Cooking Time: 15 minutes

10. Quinoa Breakfast Bowl

Ingredients:

- 1 cup cooked quinoa

- 1/4 cup unsweetened almond milk

- 1 tablespoon maple syrup or honey (optional)

- Sliced fresh fruit (e.g., peaches, berries)

- Chopped nuts (e.g., walnuts, almonds)

Instructions:

1. In a bowl, combine cooked quinoa, almond milk, and maple syrup or honey if desired.

2. Top with sliced fresh fruit and chopped nuts.

Cooking Time: 10 minutes (assuming quinoa is pre-cooked)

Leaky Gut Lunch Recipes

1. Quinoa and Grilled Vegetable Salad

Ingredients:

- 1 cup cooked quinoa

- Assorted grilled vegetables (zucchini, bell peppers, eggplant, etc.)

- Lemon-tahini dressing (lemon juice, tahini, olive oil, garlic, salt, and pepper)

Instructions:

1. Cook quinoa according to package instructions.

2. Grill the vegetables until tender.

3. Toss the quinoa and grilled vegetables with the lemon-tahini dressing.

4. Serve warm or at room temperature.

Cooking Time: 20 minutes (assuming quinoa is pre-cooked)

2. Chicken and Vegetable Stir-Fry

Ingredients:

- Boneless, skinless chicken breast, cut into strips
- Mixed vegetables (e.g., broccoli, bell peppers, carrots, snap peas)
- Stir-fry sauce (soy sauce or tamari, ginger, garlic, and honey)

Instructions:

1. Heat oil in a skillet or wok.

2. Add chicken and cook until no longer pink.

3. Add mixed vegetables and stir-fry sauce.

4. Cook until vegetables are tender and the sauce thickens.

5. Serve with cooked rice or cauliflower rice.

Cooking Time: 20 minutes

3. Lentil and Vegetable Soup

Ingredients:

- 1 cup dried green or brown lentils, rinsed and drained
- Mixed vegetables (carrots, celery, onion, etc.)
- Vegetable broth
- Seasonings (thyme, bay leaves, salt, and pepper)

Instructions:

1. In a large pot, sauté vegetables until softened.

2. Add lentils and vegetable broth.

3. Season with thyme, bay leaves, salt, and pepper.

4. Simmer until lentils are tender.

5. Remove bay leaves before serving.

Cooking Time: 45 minutes

4. Salmon and Avocado Salad

Ingredients:

- Grilled or baked salmon fillet
- Sliced avocado
- Mixcd grccns
- Lemon vinaigrette (lemon juice, olive oil, Dijon mustard, honey, salt, and pepper)

Instructions:

1. Prepare the salmon by grilling or baking until flaky.

2. Assemble the salad by placing mixed greens, avocado slices, and salmon on a plate.

3. Drizzle with lemon vinaigrette.

Cooking Time: 15-20 minutes (assuming salmon is pre-cooked)

5. Sweet Potato and Black Bean Bowl

Ingredients:

- Roasted sweet potato cubes
- Cooked black beans
- Sliced bell peppers
- Cilantro-lime dressing (lime juice, cilantro, olive oil, garlic, salt, and pepper)

Instructions:

1. Roast sweet potato cubes until tender.

2. Combine roasted sweet potatoes, black beans, and sliced bell peppers in a bowl.

3. Drizzle with cilantro-lime dressing.

Cooking Time: 30 minutes (assuming sweet potatoes are pre-roasted)

6. Turkey and Vegetable Wrap

Ingredients:

- Sliced turkey breast
- Mixed greens

- Sliced cucumber, bell peppers, and cherry tomatoes
- Gluten-free tortilla
- Hummus or avocado spread

Instructions:

1. Lay out the tortilla.

2. Spread hummus or avocado spread.

3. Layer turkey, mixed greens, and sliced vegetables.

4. Roll up and secure with toothpicks.

Cooking Time: 10 minutes

7. Zucchini Noodles with Pesto

Ingredients:

- Zucchini noodles (zoodles)
- Homemade basil pesto (basil, garlic, pine nuts, olive oil, Parmesan cheese, salt, and pepper)

Instructions:

1. Spiralize zucchini into noodles.

2. Toss zoodles with homemade basil pesto.

3. Serve chilled or at room temperature.

Cooking Time: 15 minutes

8. Tuna and Avocado Salad

Ingredients:

- Canned tuna in water, drained
- Diced avocado
- Chopped red onion
- Lemon juice, olive oil, salt, and pepper

Instructions:

1. In a bowl, combine canned tuna, diced avocado, and chopped red onion.

2. Drizzle with lemon juice and olive oil.

3. Season with salt and pepper.

4. Toss gently and serve.

Cooking Time: 10 minutes

9. Vegetable and Quinoa Stuffed Peppers

Ingredients:

- Bell peppers (red, yellow, or green)
- Cooked quinoa
- Sautéed vegetables (zucchini, carrots, spinach, etc.)
- Marinara sauce (check for added sugar)

Instructions:

1. Cut the tops off the bell peppers and remove seeds.

2. In a bowl, mix cooked quinoa and sautéed vegetables.

3. Stuff the peppers with the quinoa-vegetable mixture.

4. Place stuffed peppers in a baking dish, pour marinara sauce over them, and cover with foil.

5. Bake until peppers are tender.

Cooking Time: 45 minutes

10. Broccoli and Chicken Soup

Ingredients:

- Cooked chicken breast, shredded

- Steamed broccoli florets

- Chicken broth

- Onion, garlic, and seasonings (salt and pepper)

Instructions:

1. In a large pot, sauté onion and garlic until translucent.

2. Add chicken broth and bring to a simmer.

3. Stir in shredded chicken and steamed broccoli florets.

4. Simmer until heated through.

5. Season with salt and pepper to taste.

Cooking Time: 30 minutes (assuming chicken is pre-cooked)

CHAPTER FOUR

Leaky Gut Dinner Recipes

1. Baked Salmon with Lemon and Dill

Ingredients:

- Salmon fillets
- Fresh lemon slices
- Fresh dill
- Olive oil
- Salt and pepper

Instructions:

1. Preheat the oven to 375°F (190°C).

2. Place salmon fillets on a baking sheet lined with parchment paper.

3. Drizzle with olive oil, then season with salt and pepper.

4. Top with fresh lemon slices and dill.

5. Bake for 15-20 minutes until salmon flakes easily.

Cooking Time: 15-20 minutes

2. Roasted Chicken and Vegetables

Ingredients:

- Chicken thighs or breasts
- Assorted vegetables (carrots, bell peppers, broccoli, etc.)
- Olive oil
- Seasonings (rosemary, thyme, garlic, salt, and pepper)

Instructions:

1. Preheat the oven to 400°F (200°C).

2. Arrange chicken and vegetables on a baking sheet.

3. Drizzle with olive oil and sprinkle with seasonings.

4. Roast for about 30-35 minutes or until chicken is cooked through.

Cooking Time: 30-35 minutes

3. Sautéed Shrimp with Garlic and Spinach

Ingredients:

- Shrimp, peeled and deveined
- Fresh spinach

- Minced garlic

- Olive oil

- Lemon juice

- Red pepper flakes (optional)

- Salt and pepper

Instructions:

1. Heat olive oil in a skillet over medium heat.

2. Sauté minced garlic and red pepper flakes (if using) until fragrant.

3. Add shrimp and cook until pink.

4. Stir in fresh spinach and cook until wilted.

5. Finish with a squeeze of lemon juice, salt, and pepper.

Cooking Time: 10 minutes

4. Ground Turkey and Veggie Stir-Fry

Ingredients:

- Ground turkey

- Mixed vegetables (e.g., bell peppers, snap peas, carrots)

- Ginger and garlic (minced)

- Gluten-free soy sauce or tamari

- Sesame oil

- Salt and pepper

Instructions:

1. In a skillet, brown ground turkey until fully cooked.

2. Remove turkey and set aside.

3. In the same skillet, add sesame oil and sauté minced ginger and garlic.

4. Stir in mixed vegetables and cook until tender.

5. Return cooked turkey to the skillet, add soy sauce, and cook until heated through.

6. Season with salt and pepper.

Cooking Time: 20 minutes

5. Vegetable and Lentil Curry

Ingredients:

- Dried green or brown lentils, rinsed and drained

- Mixed vegetables (e.g., cauliflower, bell peppers, carrots, peas)

- Curry paste or powder
- Coconut milk
- Fresh cilantro for garnish (optional)

Instructions:

1. Cook lentils according to package instructions.

2. In a separate pot, sauté mixed vegetables until slightly tender.

3. Stir in curry paste or powder and cook for a few minutes.

4. Add cooked lentils and coconut milk, then simmer until vegetables are fully cooked.

5. Garnish with fresh cilantro if desired.

Cooking Time: 30 minutes

6. Baked Cod with Roasted Vegetables

Ingredients:

- Cod fillets
- Assorted vegetables (e.g., cherry tomatoes, asparagus, red onion)
- Olive oil

- Lemon zest and juice

- Fresh basil

- Salt and pepper

Instructions:

1. Preheat the oven to 375°F (190°C).

2. Place cod fillets on a baking sheet.

3. Toss vegetables with olive oil, lemon zest, salt, and pepper.

4. Arrange vegetables around the cod.

5. Drizzle lemon juice over the fish and vegetables.

6. Bake for 15-20 minutes or until the cod flakes easily.

Cooking Time: 15-20 minutes

7. Turkey and Vegetable Meatballs

Ingredients:

- Ground turkey

- Finely chopped mixed vegetables (e.g., zucchini, carrots, bell peppers)

- Fresh parsley and oregano

- Minced garlic

- Salt and pepper

- Marinara sauce (check for added sugar)

Instructions:

1. In a bowl, combine ground turkey, chopped vegetables, fresh herbs, minced garlic, salt, and pepper.

2. Form mixture into meatballs and place on a baking sheet.

3. Bake in a preheated oven at 375°F (190°C) until cooked through.

4. Serve with marinara sauce.

Cooking Time: 25-30 minutes

8. Beef and Vegetable Stir-Fry

Ingredients:

- Lean beef strips (e.g., sirloin or flank steak)

- Mixed vegetables (e.g., broccoli, snap peas, carrots)

- Stir-fry sauce (soy sauce or tamari, ginger, garlic, and honey)

- Sesame oil

- Salt and pepper

Instructions:

1. In a wok or large skillet, heat sesame oil over high heat.

2. Add beef strips and stir-fry until browned.

3. Remove beef and set aside.

4. In the same wok, stir-fry mixed vegetables.

5. Return cooked beef to the wok, add stir-fry sauce, and cook until heated through.

6. Season with salt and pepper.

Cooking Time: 20 minutes

9. Vegetable and Quinoa Stuffed Bell Peppers

Ingredients:

- Bell peppers (red, yellow, or green)
- Cooked quinoa
- Sautéed vegetables (zucchini, carrots, spinach, etc.)
- Marinara sauce (check for added sugar)

Instructions:

1. Cut the tops off the bell peppers and remove seeds.

2. In a bowl, mix cooked quinoa and sautéed vegetables.

3. Stuff the peppers with the quinoa-vegetable mixture.

4. Place stuffed peppers in a baking dish, pour marinara sauce over them, and cover with foil.

5. Bake until peppers are tender.

Cooking Time: 45 minutes

10. Chicken and Vegetable Soup

Ingredients:

- Chicken breasts or thighs
- Mixed vegetables (e.g., carrots, celery, zucchini)
- Chicken broth
- Seasonings (thyme, bay leaves, salt, and pepper)

Instructions:

1. In a large pot, sauté vegetables until softened.

2. Add chicken broth and bring to a simmer.

3. Stir in chicken and seasonings.

4. Simmer until chicken is cooked through.

5. Remove bay leaves before serving.

Cooking Time: 45 minutes

Leaky Gut Snacks Recipes

1. Greek Yogurt Parfait

Ingredients:

- 1 cup Greek yogurt (if tolerated)
- 1/2 cup fresh berries (e.g., blueberries, strawberries)
- 1 tablespoon honey or maple syrup (optional)
- 2 tablespoons chopped nuts (e.g., almonds, walnuts)

Instructions:

1. In a glass or bowl, layer Greek yogurt, berries, and a drizzle of honey or maple syrup if desired.

2. Sprinkle with chopped nuts on top.

Preparation Time: 5 minutes

2. Guacamole with Veggie Sticks

Ingredients:

- 2 ripe avocados
- 1 tomato, diced
- 1/4 cup diced red onion
- 1/4 cup chopped cilantro
- Juice of 1 lime
- Salt and pepper to taste
- Carrot, cucumber, and bell pepper sticks for dipping

Instructions:

1. Mash avocados in a bowl.

2. Stir in diced tomato, red onion, cilantro, and lime juice.

3. Season with salt and pepper.

4. Serve with vegetable sticks.

Preparation Time: 10 minutes

3. Almond Butter and Banana Slices

Ingredients:

- 1 ripe banana
- 2 tablespoons almond butter
- A drizzle of honey (optional)

Instructions:

1. Slice the banana into rounds.

2. Spread almond butter on each banana slice.

3. Drizzle with honey if desired.

Preparation Time: 5 minutes

4. Mixed Berry Smoothie

Ingredients:

- 1 cup mixed berries (e.g., blueberries, raspberries, strawberries)
- 1/2 cup Greek yogurt (if tolerated) or dairy-free yogurt
- 1/2 cup almond milk
- 1 tablespoon honey or maple syrup (optional)

Instructions:

1. Blend mixed berries, Greek yogurt (if using), almond milk, and honey or maple syrup until smooth.

2. Pour into a glass and enjoy.

Preparation Time: 5 minutes

5. Chia Seed Pudding

Ingredients:

- 2 tablespoons chia seeds
- 1 cup almond milk (or any preferred milk)
- 1/2 teaspoon vanilla extract
- Fresh fruit (e.g., sliced bananas, berries) for topping

Instructions:

1. In a jar or bowl, mix chia seeds, almond milk, and vanilla extract.

2. Stir well and refrigerate overnight.

3. In the morning, top with fresh fruit before serving.

Preparation Time: 5 minutes (plus overnight soaking)

6. Hummus with Veggie Dippers

Ingredients:

- Hummus (homemade or store-bought)
- Sliced cucumber, carrot sticks, and bell pepper strips

Instructions:

1. Arrange sliced vegetables on a plate.

2. Serve with a bowl of hummus for dipping.

Preparation Time: 5 minutes

7. Baked Sweet Potato Fries

Ingredients:

- Sweet potatoes, cut into strips
- Olive oil
- Paprika, garlic powder, salt, and pepper

Instructions:

1. Preheat the oven to 425°F (220°C).

2. Toss sweet potato strips with olive oil, paprika, garlic powder, salt, and pepper.

3. Arrange on a baking sheet and bake until crispy, flipping halfway through.

Preparation Time: 30 minutes

8. Rice Cakes with Avocado

Ingredients:

- Rice cakes (gluten-free if necessary)
- Ripe avocado
- Salt, pepper, and red pepper flakes (optional)

Instructions:

1. Slice ripe avocado and mash it lightly.

2. Spread mashed avocado on rice cakes.

3. Season with salt, pepper, and red pepper flakes if desired.

Preparation Time: 5 minutes

9. Mixed Nuts and Dried Fruits

Ingredients:

- Mixed nuts (e.g., almonds, walnuts, cashews)
- Dried fruits (e.g., raisins, apricots, cranberries)

Instructions:

1. Combine mixed nuts and dried fruits in a bowl.

2. Portion into small snack-sized bags for easy grab-and-go.

Preparation Time: 5 minutes

10. Veggie Sushi Rolls

Ingredients:

- Nori seaweed sheets
- Cooked sushi rice
- Sliced cucumber, avocado, and bell pepper
- Soy sauce or tamari for dipping

Instructions:

1. Lay a sheet of nori on a bamboo sushi mat.

2. Spread a thin layer of sushi rice over the nori, leaving a small border.

3. Place slices of cucumber, avocado, and bell pepper in the center.

4. Roll the nori tightly, wetting the edges to seal.

5. Slice into bite-sized pieces.

6. Serve with soy sauce or tamari for dipping.

Preparation Time: 20 minutes

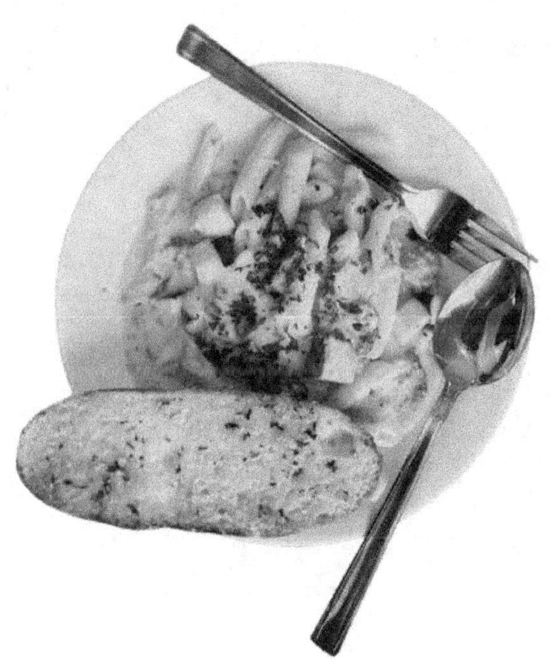

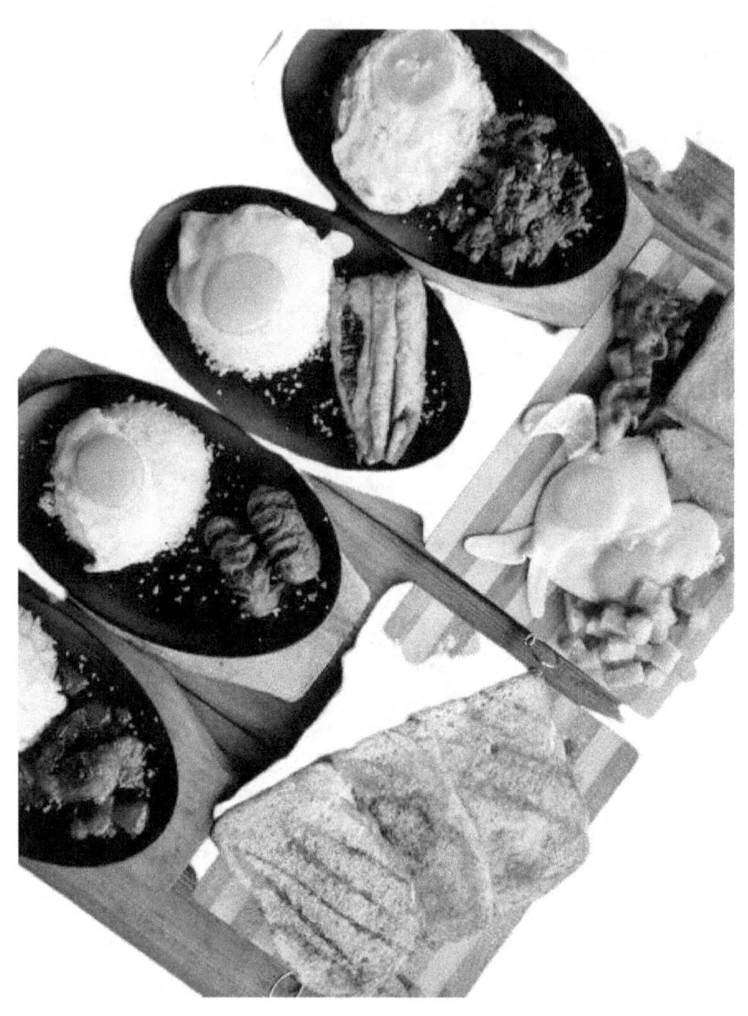

CONCLUSION

The leaky gut diet plays a crucial role in supporting gut health and overall well-being for individuals suffering from leaky gut syndrome. This dietary approach prioritizes the consumption of foods that can promote gut healing, reduce inflammation, and alleviate symptoms associated with this condition.

The leaky gut diet emphasizes the inclusion of whole, unprocessed foods rich in fiber, vitamins, and minerals. These foods not only provide essential nutrients but also support the growth of beneficial gut bacteria, which are integral to maintaining a healthy intestinal lining.

Furthermore, the diet promotes the consumption of anti-inflammatory foods like fatty fish (rich in omega-3 fatty acids), colorful fruits and vegetables (packed with antioxidants), and herbs and spices (such as turmeric and ginger), which have been shown to reduce inflammation and promote gut health.

Moreover, by eliminating or reducing foods known to contribute to gut irritation, such as refined sugars, artificial additives, processed foods, and potentially allergenic ingredients, individuals with leaky gut syndrome can significantly improve their digestive health.

Probiotic-rich foods and supplements also have a vital role in the leaky gut diet. These sources of beneficial bacteria can help restore a balanced gut microbiome, which is essential for a healthy intestinal lining.

In conclusion, the leaky gut diet is a well-rounded approach that combines nutrition, lifestyle, and mindful eating to support and promote gut health. By adopting this diet and making informed food choices, individuals with leaky gut syndrome can take significant steps toward healing their gut and improving their overall quality of life.

However, it's crucial to remember that consistency and patience are key, and the best results often come with a holistic approach that includes stress management, adequate sleep, and regular physical activity in addition to a balanced diet.